THE WHOLE BODY RESET FOR WEIGHT LOSS MANAGEMENT

Transform your health, energy and 30-days Meal prep recipes to Unlock Your Metabolism and Ignite Lasting Change.

ALLEN A CARY

Table of contents

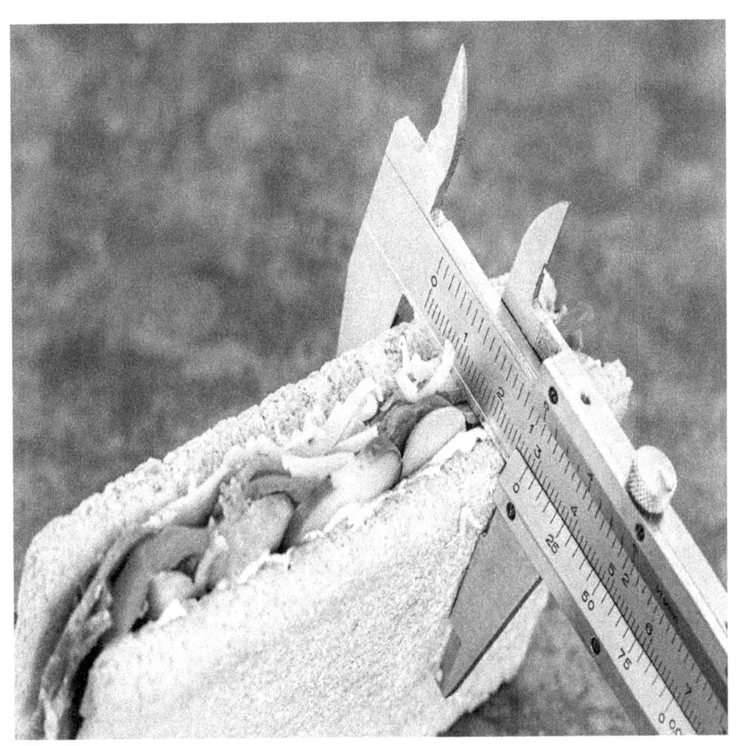

@2023 by [Allen A. Cary] Copyright

Each of the rights reserved Except for brief quotations included in critical reviews and specific additional noncommercial uses allowed by copyright law, no part of this book may be reproduced, stored in a retrieval system, or passed in any form or by any method, whether electronic, mechanical, photocopying, recording, or otherwise.

INTRODUCTION

Are you fed up with calorie counting nonstop, yo-yo dieting, and the depressing feeling that comes from watching the scale's number stay the same? Are you yearning for a weight reduction solution that really resets your body and mind for long-lasting improvement, something that goes beyond restriction and fast fixes? If yes, welcome to The Whole Body Reset—your road map to discovering a happier, healthier version of yourself. This book is about more than simply losing weight, but it's a pretty fantastic side effect. It's an opportunity to completely reset the system, do away with the antiquated guidelines, and adopt a holistic weight-management strategy.

Forget what you believe to be true about dieting. Calorie charts and stringent meal planning are going out of style. Rather, we'll explore the little-known science of hormones, metabolism, and the benefits of attentive eating. You'll discover why conventional diets often backfire and how to feed your body with wholesome, delectable foods that energize every cell and unleash your body's innate ability to burn fat.

This reset is much more than just the plate. We'll discuss how important it is to exercise, get enough sleep, and manage your stress if you want to lose weight. You'll learn how to tame the stress beast that might impede your development, prioritize good sleep, and include activity that you genuinely love.

However, this goes beyond a simple bodily change. We'll also explore the critical mentality adjustment for long-term success. You'll discover how to overcome negative behaviors, develop self-compassion, and appreciate each step along the way.

This book will accompany you on a unique journey to become a healthier, lighter, and more energetic version of yourself. Disregard short-term remedies and passing trends. This is about designing a sustainable way of living that you will really like.

So grab a seat, prepare to let go of your emotional and physical belongings, and press the reset button on your life. It's time to give your body and mind the tools they need to finally attain your health goals rather than merely hoping for it.

Chapter 1: Why You Need a Whole Body Reset for Weight Loss

There are a lot of people who are solely focused on certain diets, workout routines, or current weight loss pills in their efforts to achieve their weight elimination objectives. On the other hand, a holistic approach, sometimes known as a "whole body reset," can frequently be the most effective and durable methodology for weight reduction. A complete approach to weight reduction will be addressed in this chapter, with an emphasis placed on the linked nature of the many body systems. The reasons for the need of such a strategy are discussed.

1. Acquiring an Understanding of the Close Relationships Within the Body

A complex and delicately integrated network of organs, hormones, and metabolic processes, the human body is a complex and tightly woven system. The processes of gaining and losing weight are not independent occurrences but rather are impacted by a wide range of variables, such as one's food, level of physical activity, amount of sleep, stress levels, and general health. It is possible to get less-than-ideal outcomes and experience frustration on the path to weight reduction if one disregards the linked nature of these components.

2. Taking Action to Address the Root Causes

Counting calories or engaging in vigorous physical activity routines are two methods that often fail to address the underlying factors that lead to weight gain. In order to reset the whole body, it is necessary to identify and treat the underlying problems that are causing the problem, such as hormone imbalances, dietary deficiencies, and unhealthy lifestyle behaviors. By targeting these core reasons, people may develop a foundation for lasting weight reduction and general well-being.

3. Breaking the Cycle of Yo-Yo Dieting

Many people fall into the trap of yo-yo dieting, which is when they experience short-term weight reduction followed by regaining weight. This loop may be damaging to both physical and mental health. A whole body reset tries to interrupt this tendency by fostering long-term lifestyle adjustments that promote weight management and general health.

4. Optimizing Metabolism and Energy Balance

A thorough approach to weight management entails improving the body's metabolism and creating a healthy energy balance. This goes beyond the typical emphasis on calorie restriction and hard exercise. By examining elements like nutrition timing, meal structure, and metabolic health, people may boost their body's capacity to burn fat and maintain a healthy weight.

5. Achieving Mind-Body Balance

The relationship between the mind and body plays a significant role in weight control. Stress, emotional eating, and poor mental health might hamper weight reduction attempts. A whole body reset involves tactics to attain mind-body balance, including practices of mindfulness, methods for reducing stress, and psychological well-being.

6. Setting the Stage for Lasting Change

In essence, a whole body reset is not just a short-term answer but a comprehensive and lasting strategy to weight reduction. By treating the linked aspects of the body, recognising fundamental causes, and cultivating mind-body harmony, people may set the foundation for enduring evolution and begin on a path towards a healthier, more satisfying life. This book will walk you through the ideas and techniques required to commence an effective whole body reset for weight reduction.

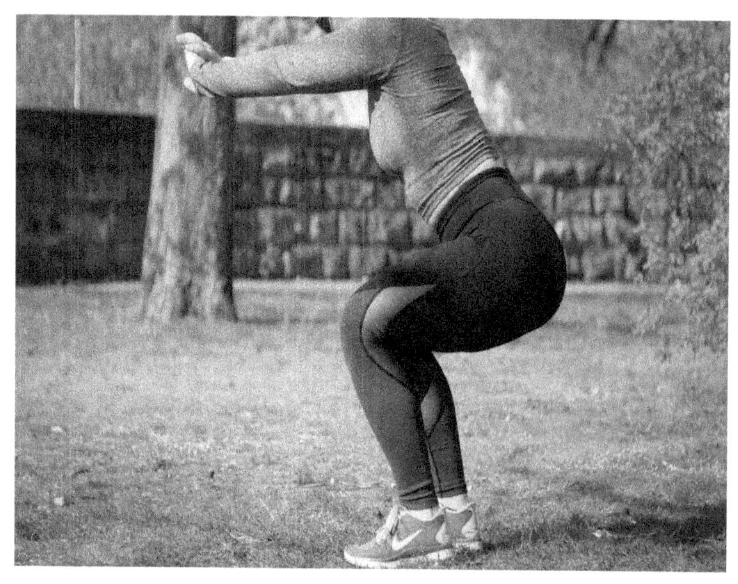

Chapter 2: Unveiling the Hidden Culprits: Physiology, Habits, and Mindset

exposing the mysteries behind our actions in the maze of human behavior requires a comprehension of the complex interactions between physiology, habits, and mindset. This chapter seeks to expose the unseen wrongdoers who mold our everyday decisions and affect how our lives unfold.

First Section: Physiology

Our actions are greatly influenced by the intricate network of organs and systems that make up the human body. Our physiological responses impact our behavior in both visible and invisible ways. Examples include the subtle release of dopamine during moments of joy and the surge of adrenaline in response to stress. By investigating the physiological foundations of our behavior, we can reveal the silent orchestrator operating behind the scenes.

The complex dance of hormones, neurotransmitters, and physiological processes that influences our ability to make decisions is covered in this section. We can better understand why some behaviors are ingrained in our biology by delving into the physiological aspects. This knowledge can also enable us to alter our behavior for the better.

Second Section: Habits

Our daily actions are greatly influenced by our habits, which are those automatic behaviors ingrained in our lives. Our lives are shaped by our habits, whether they are the daily routines we follow or the subconscious ways we react to stressors. In order to shed light on the neural pathways that give habits their resilience, this section looks at the psychology of habit formation.

We have the ability to effect change if we comprehend how habits are formed. Readers are provided with a roadmap to change their daily routines and, in turn, their lives, by exploring strategies for fostering positive habits and breaking detrimental ones.

Third Section: Mindset

Our attitude and reactions are shaped by our mindset, which serves as a filter through which we view the world. While resilience and success can be sparked by a growth mindset, a fixed mindset may impede personal development. This section examines how behavior is influenced by mindset and how developing an optimistic and flexible mindset can significantly alter one's circumstances.

Readers are encouraged to reflect on and alter their own mindsets through psychological insights and examples from real life. A mindset that is supportive of long-term goal achievement, resilience, and personal growth is fostered through useful exercises and advice.

We take a tour through the complex relationships that exist between mindset, habits, and physiology in this chapter. We create the foundation for a profound investigation of self-awareness and personal growth by exposing the hidden villains influencing our behavior.

Chapter 3: Setting Sustainable Goals: Beyond the Number on the Scale

In our pursuit of a life that is both healthier and more satisfying, it is of the greatest significance that we become aware of the fact that real well-being encompasses a great deal more than the simple numbers that show up on a scale. Although one's weight might serve as a measure of their overall health, it is just one component of a far more comprehensive and elaborate picture.

In this chapter, we will discuss the notion of creating sustainable objectives that exceed beyond the constraints of the scale, with a center of attention on holistic well-being and success over the long term.

1. Adopting a Holistic Approach to Wellness

There is more than one facet to the idea of wellness. It takes into account many aspects of our existence, such as our physical, mental, emotional, and social well-being along with other aspects. When we set out on our journey to adopt a healthy way of life, it is crucial that we take into consideration all of these components. Rather than focusing exclusively on weight reduction, sustainable objectives should include the overarching objective of improving their entire wellbeing.

2. Defining Personal Success

Success is a subjective notion, and each individual's definition will change. Instead of following conventional conventions or arbitrary criteria, it's vital to establish what success means to you individually. This may involve attaining a specific degree of fitness, building mental resilience, or creating healthy connections. Adapt your objectives so that they are in line with your own desires.

3. Establishing Realistic Milestones

A common cause of dissatisfaction and exhaustion is setting objectives that are impossible to achieve. Break down your ambitions into simple, attainable stages. Celebrate minor triumphs along the way, rewarding healthy behavior and drive. This progressive strategy not only makes the trip more sustainable but also boosts the chance of long-term success.

4. Cultivating Healthy Habits

Rather than fixating on short-term achievements, underscore the creation of enduring behaviors. Focus on adding healthy meals, frequent physical exercise, and mindfulness into your daily routine. Building the basis of healthy behaviors develops a sustained commitment to well-being, overcoming the ephemeral nature of fad diets or intensive training regimens.

5. Monitoring Non-Scale Victories

Look beyond the scale for indicators of progress. Non-scale successes, such as better energy levels, improved sleep, enhanced mood, and better self-esteem, give a more thorough sense of your well-being. Acknowledge and appreciate these victories as they contribute greatly to your overall health journey.

6. Building a Support System

Surround yourself with a supporting environment that promotes and uplifts you. Share your objectives with friends, family, or join groups that coincide with your aims. Having a solid support system not only promotes accountability but also gives important encouragement during hard times.

7. Practicing Self-Compassion

Recognize that setbacks are a normal part of any endeavor. Approach obstacles with self-compassion, realizing that perfection is unattainable. Learn from failures, change your objectives if required, and continue pushing ahead with a positive perspective.

By moving our attention from the restrictive boundaries of the scale to a more holistic and sustainable strategy, we pave the road for permanent well-being. This chapter encourages you to reframe success, establish realistic objectives, create good habits, recognise non-scale accomplishments, build a solid support system, and cultivate compassion for themselves. Together, these principles will lead you towards a rewarding and sustainable route to a better, happier life.

Chapter 4: Fueling for Function: Nutrition Principles for Reset & Beyond

We will explore the fundamentals of nutrition in this chapter, which are critical to maintaining optimum performance and helping your body reset. Reaching your wellness and health aims requires knowing how to provide your body with the proper nutrition.

1. The Basis:

Foods High in Nutrients
Eating foods high in nutrients is the cornerstone of a healthy diet. Fruits, vegetables, whole grains, lean meats, and good fats are a few of them. You can make sure that your body gets a wide variety of vitamins, minerals, and other essential components that are required for general health by making these foods a priority.

2.   Maintaining   Macronutrient Balance:

Sustaining a balanced diet of macronutrients—fats, proteins, and carbohydrates—is essential for proper body function and long-term energy. Gaining an improved awareness of your own requirements and modifying the proportions of these macronutrients will help you perform better, recover more quickly, and maintain better metabolic health.

3. Drinking Enough Water for Health:

Drinking enough water is crucial for resetting your body, yet it's sometimes disregarded. Numerous biological processes, including digestion, nutrition absorption, and controlling the temperature, depend on water. Develop practices that promote ideal fluid balance and educate yourself about your particular hydration requirements.

4. **Timing Is Important:** Frequency and Meal Planning

Your energy levels and metabolism may be affected by the times you eat meals and snacks. Examine meal planning and frequency techniques that fit your objectives and lifestyle. Learn how timing your nutrients may help you perform better, recover more quickly, and feel better overall.

5. Nutraceuticals and Functional Foods:

There are certain foods and substances that may help you on your health path even more. Examine the function of functional meals and determine when taking pills can be helpful. But it's crucial to use care when supplementing and give priority to getting your nutrients from real meals whenever you can.

6. Customizing Your Method:

It is important to acknowledge that dietary needs differ throughout people. Dietary needs depend on a number of factors, including age, gender, activity level, and health. Customize your dietary strategy to fit your particular demands and keep an eye out for changes in your body.

7. Overcoming Difficulties:

Emotional Consumption and Social Factors

Long-term success calls for tackling the psychological components of diet. Discover how to handle social settings, stop emotional eating, and have a healthy relationship with food. Maintaining good eating habits requires cultivating a resilient attitude.

8. Observing and Modifying:

Sustained success requires regular assessment of how you are doing and modification of your dietary strategy. You may make educated judgments and modify your dietary plan by being aware of your body's signals, whether via monitoring metrics, evaluating how your body feels, or consulting a specialist.

We've gone over the basic dietary fundamentals in this chapter, which will help you through your reset and beyond. You'll create a strong basis for long-term health and wellbeing by accepting these ideas and modifying them to fit your own requirements.

Chapter 5: Bye-Bye Processed, Hello Whole: The Reset Food Guide

inevitably embark out on a life-changing journey towards a healthier and more energetic lifestyle in this crucial chapter. Say goodbye for producing meals and welcome the healing power of whole, unprocessed substances. Your compass on this thrilling journey towards regeneration is the Reset Food Guide.

Taking Up Whole Foods

Whole foods maintain their inherent deliciousness and nutritional integrity since they are neither refined or processed. As the primary source of crucial vitamins, minerals, and nutrients in their purest form, they constitute the foundation of a reenergized diet.

The Potency of Plant-Based

Turn your attention to foods that are plant-based and high in fiber, antioxidants, and phytonutrients. Nuts, legumes, fruits, and vegetables that are in season become your partners in fostering general health and longevity.

Complete Grains for Long-Term Energy

Exchange refined grains for their whole equivalents. Processed grains just are insufficient to the long-lasting energy, fiber, and health benefits of brown rice, quinoa, and oats.

Using the Reset Dietary Guide

The List of Green Lights

Find a plethora of meals that are approved for your Reset journey. These involve complete grains, lean proteins, healthy fats, and fresh fruit. When organizing your meals, use this list as a reference.

Take Care with Yellow Light Foods

When it comes to meals in the yellow light category, use discretion. These may contain junk food with little nutritional content, but they are not forbidden. Pay attention to frequency and portion sizes.

Red light: Move cautiously

These are the foods that need to be eaten in moderation. Sugary, highly processed snacks and drinks belong in this group. Realizing how these decisions will affect you is essential to a good reset.

Reset Your Success Recipes

wholesome breakfast

Smoothie bowls, avocado toast, and overnight oats are a few healthy ways to start your day. These dishes provide a happy mood for the day.

Plant-Based Lunches

Discover the colorful world of vegetarian wraps, grain bowls, and salads. These plant-based meals supply your body the nourishment it needs to function better, giving you more energy and clarity.

Suppertime Sweets
With recipes like roasted veggies, grilled lean meats, and whole-grain meals, dinner becomes a fascinating culinary adventure. Rekindle your love of cooking and eating healthful food.

Maintaining the Reset Way of Life
Mastering Meal Preparation

Your secret weapon for sticking to the Reset lifestyle is effective food preparation. Make sure you always have healthful alternatives on hand by batch cooking whole meals.

Conscientious Consumption
Make eating a conscious activity. Take note of your body's signals of hunger and fullness, enjoy the flavors, and recognise the nutrition that comes from eating entire foods.

Honor advancements

Celebrate and give thanks for the improvements you've made. Every step you take towards your Reset journey is a victory, whether it's more energy, a happier mood, or better overall wellbeing.

Goodbye, processed, and hello, entire! With the help of the Reset Food Guide, you can make wise choices that are healthy- that pave the way for a refreshed and rejuvenated you. Accept the adventure, enjoy the tastes, and bask in the bright vitality that whole meals provide.

Chapter 6: Meal Magic: Delicious & Nutritious Recipes for Your Reset

Greetings and welcome to the Meal Magic chapter, where we will delve into a range of delectable and nourishing foods that may assist in resetting your mind and body. These dishes are meant to satisfy your cravings, nourish your body, and provide vital nutrients. Together, we will go on a gastronomic adventure that will satisfy your cravings for healthful, tasty food while also providing nourishment for your body.

See what's in planned for you:

Breakfast Bliss: Invigorate your senses and energize your body with colorful smoothies, fluffy frittatas, and protein-rich porridge bowls.

Lightness at Lunch: Light and fulfilling salads full of color and texture, hearty soups that soothe your soul, and veggie-and protein-rich wraps are great ways to beat the noon slump.

Suppertime Treats: Enjoy delicious stir-fries, one-pan miracles, and slow-cooked masterpieces that will awaken your senses and give you a boost of energy for your evening meals.

Solutions for Snack Attacks: Replace manufactured junk food with wholesome options that will satisfy your desires without impeding your progress, such as protein muffins, vegetable dips, and homemade energy snacks.

Sweet Contentment: Enjoy naturally sweetened sweets such as chia seed pudding, baked apples and rich dark chocolate mousse without feeling guilty.

But this is more than simply a cookbook. There are useful recommendations accompanying each dish:

Substitute ingredients to suit your dietary requirements and tastes in the recipes.

Time-saving tips: Prepare wholesome meals quickly, even on hectic workdays.

Highlights of nutrition: Recalibrate your objectives and learn how each element affects your general health.

Prepare to:

Give up the diet mindset and enjoy cooking with genuine, fresh ingredients and the ability of food to nourish your body from the inside out.

Taste new flavors: Take culinary risks by experimenting with unusual flavor combos, unique spices, and influences from across the world.

Give your body what it needs to succeed: Consume food for optimum health, energy, and performance to make sure that taste fuels your reset journey.

Now put on your apron, widen your mind, and let's unleash the magic of mealtime!

Recipe 1: Quinoa Power Bowl

Ingredients:

1 cup quinoa, rinsed

2 cups water

1 cup cherry tomatoes, halved

1 cucumber, diced

1 cup cooked chickpeas

1/2 cup feta cheese, crumbled

1/4 cup red onion, finely chopped

2 tablespoons olive oil

2 tablespoons lemon juice

Salt and pepper to taste

Fresh parsley for garnish

Instructions:

Cook quinoa according to package instructions. Once cooked, fluff it with a fork and let it cool.

In a large bowl, combine the quinoa, cherry tomatoes, cucumber, chickpeas, feta cheese, and red onion.

In a small bowl, whisk together olive oil, lemon juice, salt, and pepper.

Pour the dressing over the quinoa mixture and toss gently to combine.

Garnish with fresh parsley before serving. This Quinoa Power Bowl is not

only colorful but also packed with
protein and vitamins.

Recipe 2: Salmon Avocado Salad

Ingredients:

2 salmon filets

4 cups mixed salad greens

1 avocado, sliced

1 cup cherry tomatoes, halved

1/4 cup red bell pepper, thinly sliced

2 tablespoons balsamic vinaigrette

Salt and pepper to taste

Lemon wedges for serving

Instructions:

Season the salmon filets with salt and pepper. Grill or bake until cooked through.

In a large bowl, combine the mixed salad greens, sliced avocado, cherry tomatoes, and red bell pepper.

Place the grilled salmon on top of the salad.

Drizzle the balsamic vinaigrette over the salad and salmon.

Serve with lemon wedges for an extra burst of flavor. This Salmon Avocado

Salad is a nutrient-packed meal that's both satisfying and delicious.

Recipe 3: Berry Bliss Smoothie

Ingredients:

1 cup mixed berries (strawberries, blueberries, raspberries)

1 banana, peeled

1/2 cup Greek yogurt

1 cup almond milk

1 tablespoon honey

Ice cubes (optional)

Instructions:

In a blender, combine mixed berries, banana, Greek yogurt, almond milk, and honey.

Blend until smooth. Add ice cubes if desired and blend again.

Pour the smoothie into a glass and enjoy this Berry Bliss Smoothie that's rich in antioxidants and vitamins.

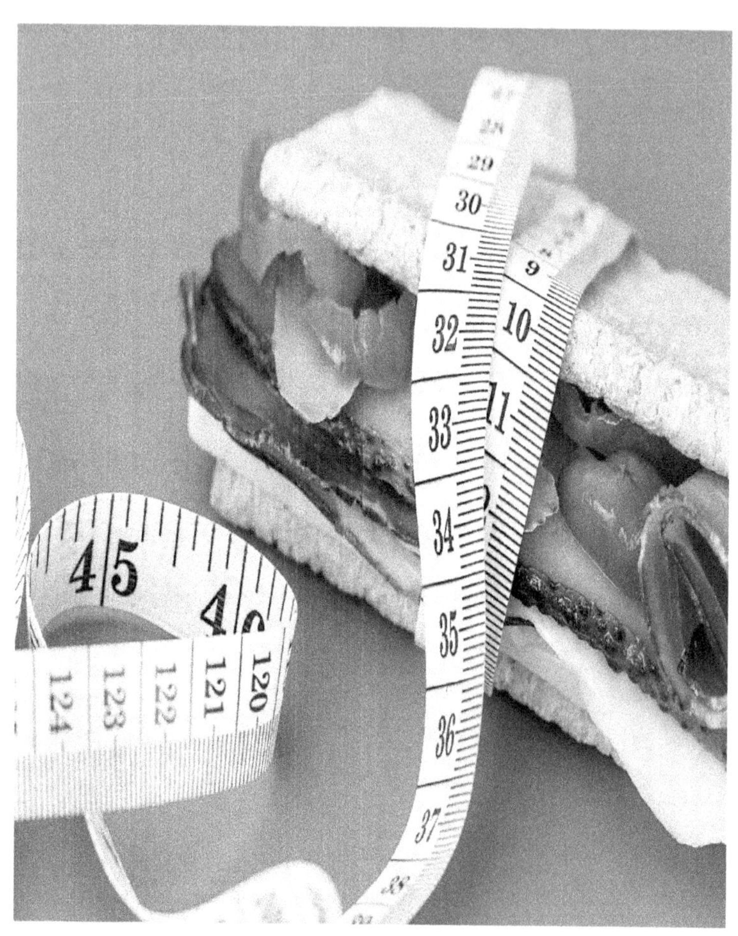

Chapter 7: Mindful Munching: Overcoming Emotional Eating & Building a Healthy Relationship with Food

In this chapter, we will dig in the key element that is mindful munching, concentrating on conquering emotional eating and creating an appealing and healthy connection with food. A healthy diet and attaining general well-being may be significantly hampered by emotional eating. By developing mindfulness in what you eat, you may create a closer relationship with your body, detect emotional triggers, and make intentional choices that promote your health and happiness.

Section 1: An Overview of Emotional Consumption

- ***What Emotional Eating Is About:***

Examine the idea of emotionally driven eating and how it affects general health.

Understand the distinction between emotional and physical hunger.

Detecting Emotional Stressors:

Talk about typical emotional causes that lead to overeating.

Promote introspection to identify one's own triggers.

Section 2: Techniques for Mindful Eating

- *The Craft of Conscious Eating:*

Describe the advantages of mindful eating and its guiding principles.

Point out how important it is to be present while eating.

- *Using Your Senses:*

Examine how eating mindfully is enhanced when you use all five senses. Offer hands-on activities to develop sensory awareness.

Section 3: Establishing a Salubrious Bond with Food

- *Dismissing the Diet Mentality*

Talk about the negative effects of rigid diets and the significance of taking a comprehensive approach.
Promote the transition from a constructive way of thinking to a sustainable, well-rounded strategy.

- *Sensual Consumption:*

Explain the idea of eating intuitively and paying attention to your body's cues.
Give advice on how to get back in touch with your body's natural hunger and fullness signals.

Section 4: Useful Techniques for Mindful Eating

- *Maintaining a Nutrition Log:*

Encourage keeping a food diary to record eating habits and feelings.

Give advice on the proper usage of a food journal.

Establishing a Help Network:

Stress the importance of a network or community of support in promoting a healthy diet.
Provide advice on how to create and manage a trustworthy support network.

Chapter 8: Movement Matters: Exercise Choices for Every Fitness Level

This chapter explores the significance of movement and examines a range of exercise regimens appropriate for people of all fitness levels. This chapter gives helpful advice on creating a customized workout programme, regardless of your level of expertise or desire for new challenges. It is ideal for beginners starting out on the path to a more active lifestyle.

1. Recognising the Importance of Motion

Prior to getting into certain exercises, it's important to know why movement is important. Frequent exercise has several advantages, including better mood and cognitive performance as well as weight control and cardiovascular health improvements. To ensure long-term devotion to your fitness quest, the secret is to choose things you like.

2. Adapting Exercises to Your Degree of Fitness a Novices

Begin with low-impact exercises like cycling, swimming, or walking if you're new to exercising. Introduce strength training gradually by starting with bodyweight activities like push-ups and squats. This preparatory stage prepares the body for more strenuous exercise. If you've had some experience working out, switch up your regimen. Combine weight training with cardio activities like dance or jogging. If you want to keep things interesting and difficult, think about taking fitness programmes or joining a sports team. Fitness aficionados with experience may push their limits even further. Robust bodyweight exercises, advanced weightlifting, and vigorous interval training (HIIT) are all great options. Concentrate on perfecting your form and learning about specialized training techniques.

3. Choosing Pleasurable Activities

The secret to maintaining a regular exercise routine is to choose activities you really like. Try out various sports, yoga, and martial arts, among other things. You're more likely to continue with your exercises if you look forward to them.

4. Including Mobility and Flexibility

Despite your fitness level, don't forget flexibility and mobility workouts. These exercises, which include dynamic stretching and yoga, enhance joint range of motion and reduce the risk of injury, thereby encouraging general well-being.

5. Establishing a Harmonious Schedule

Exercises combining cardiovascular, strength, flexibility, and balance make up a well-rounded fitness programme. Make sure to include a comprehensive approach to training while customizing your programme to meet what you want and interests.

6. Making Safe Progress

Put safety first as you continue on your fitness adventure. In order to avert excessive exercise and lower the chance of injury, gradually raise the level of difficulty and tension. Pay attention to your body, and don't be afraid to seek advice from fitness experts.

Chapter 9: Sleep Sanctuary: Rest & Recharge for Optimal Health

The caliber of our sleep is one of the most important, but sometimes disregarded, factors in the quest of optimum health. Sleep is an essential process that enables our bodies and brains to rejuvenate, heal, and be ready for the demands of the next day.

It is not only a time for relaxation. Establishing a sleep sanctuary is crucial to guaranteeing a favorable atmosphere that encourages deep, revitalizing sleep.

The Value of Restful Sleep:

Prior to exploring the components of a sleep sanctuary, let us emphasize the importance of getting good sleep. The significant effects of sleep on mental health, physical health, and cognitive performance have been shown in several research. A greater likelihood of chronic illnesses including obesity, diabetes, and cardiovascular diseases is linked to inadequate sleep.

Additionally, it may affect one's mood, focus, and ability to make decisions.

A Sleep Sanctuary's Essentials: Cozy Mattress and Pillows

Purchasing comfortable pillows and mattresses is essential. Your bed is the cornerstone of your sleeping haven, so selecting a mattress and pillows that provide enough support may greatly improve the quality of your sleep.

Light Control:

Limit your exposure to light to create a sleep-friendly atmosphere. To filter out outside light, think about using blackout curtains or blinds.

Furthermore, avoid using blue-light-emitting electronics just before bed since this kind of light might disrupt the body's melatonin synthesis.

Temperature Regulation:

It's critical to keep your body temperature at the ideal level for sleeping. For the majority of individuals, a cool environment with a temperature of around 60–67 degrees Fahrenheit (15–20 degrees Celsius) is advised. Try different clothes and bedding combinations to see what keeps you pleasantly cool.

Declutter Your Space:

Being unable to relax in your bedroom due to clutter and disarray may lead to tension and worry. Preserve your sleeping haven neat and clear of any unneeded distractions.

Calm Colors & The decor:

For your bedroom's decoration, go with neutral, calming hues. Earth tones, gentle blues, and greens may all help to create a peaceful ambiance. Think about including calming components like artwork or plants.

Reduce the amount of distracting noise in the place where you sleep. To reduce noise and create a calmer environment, you may use earplugs, white noise devices, or relaxing music.

Create a Calm Night Habit:

Create a routine before bed to let your body know when it's time to relax. This might include engaging in relaxing activities like deep breathing, reading, or light stretching.

Limit Screen Time:

Because blue light from electronics may disrupt your circadian cycle, try to limit your time spent in front of a screen before bed. Try to avoid using screens for at least one hour preceding going to bed.

Constructing a sleep sanctuary requires deliberate decisions and modifications to your bedroom setup and nightly schedule. Making sleep a priority not only improves your physical health but also has a good effect on your general well-being and day-to-day functioning. Recall that investing in a well-designed sleep sanctuary may significantly improve your long-term health and vigor.

Chapter 10: Stress Reset: Tools & Techniques for Calm & Clarity

Stress has become an inevitable aspect of our lives in this fast-paced, high-demanding environment. Stress may negatively impact our emotional and physical health, regardless of the source—workplace demands, personal difficulties, or outside influences. Fortunately, there are practical tools and methods available to help us reset our stress levels and regain clarity and serenity. We'll look at a number of techniques in this chapter that may assist you in controlling your life and stress.

Section 1: Techniques for Breathing

- **Inhaling deeply**

Discover how to rapidly relax your nervous system by practicing deep breathing. Examine several deep breathing techniques that you may use in your everyday life to lower stress and improve awareness.

- **Breathing in a Box**

Learn the benefits of box breathing, a method that athletes and professionals utilize to improve concentration and lower anxiety. For the most effective way to relieve stress, practise box breathing by following a step-by-step method.

Section 2: Meditation with Mindfulness

- **Mindful Awareness**

Examine the idea of mindfulness and the ways you might incorporate it into your everyday activities. Discover easy mindfulness meditation methods to focus your attention on the here and now, promoting mental clarity and serenity.

- **Directed Introspection**

Discover the advantages of guided meditation, as trained teachers take you through relaxing and centering sessions. Choose the best guided meditation that suits your requirements and tastes.

Section 3: Exercise

- **Yoga as a Stress-Reduction Technique**

Explore the relationship between yoga and stress reduction. Discover easy-to-learn yoga postures and sequences that enhance balance and relaxation while enhancing both mental and physical health.

- **Exercise for Cardiovascular Health**

Recognise how cardiovascular exercise impacts the chemicals that cause stress. Find pleasant pursuits that raise your heart rate and relieve accumulated stress.

Section 4: Mental Methods

- **Restructuring Cognitive Processes**

Cognitive restructuring may be used to question and refute harmful thinking processes. Discover how to recognise and alter negative ideas that add to your stress.

- **Clarity Through Journaling**

Accept the healing potential of journaling. Express your ideas and feelings via writing to identify stressors and come up with workable solutions.

Section 5: Modifications to Lifestyle

- **Good Sleep Practices**

Examine the relationship between stress and sleep. Adopt sensible sleep hygiene procedures to guarantee revitalizing and regenerative sleep, which enhances general wellbeing.

- **Organizing Your Time**

Develop your time management skills to boost productivity and lessen overwhelm. Learn how to set priorities for your work and make a balanced daily plan.

You may reset your stress levels and cultivate clarity and calmness in the face of life's obstacles by implementing these tools and practices into your daily routine. Investigate the tactics described in this chapter to start living a more robust and balanced life.

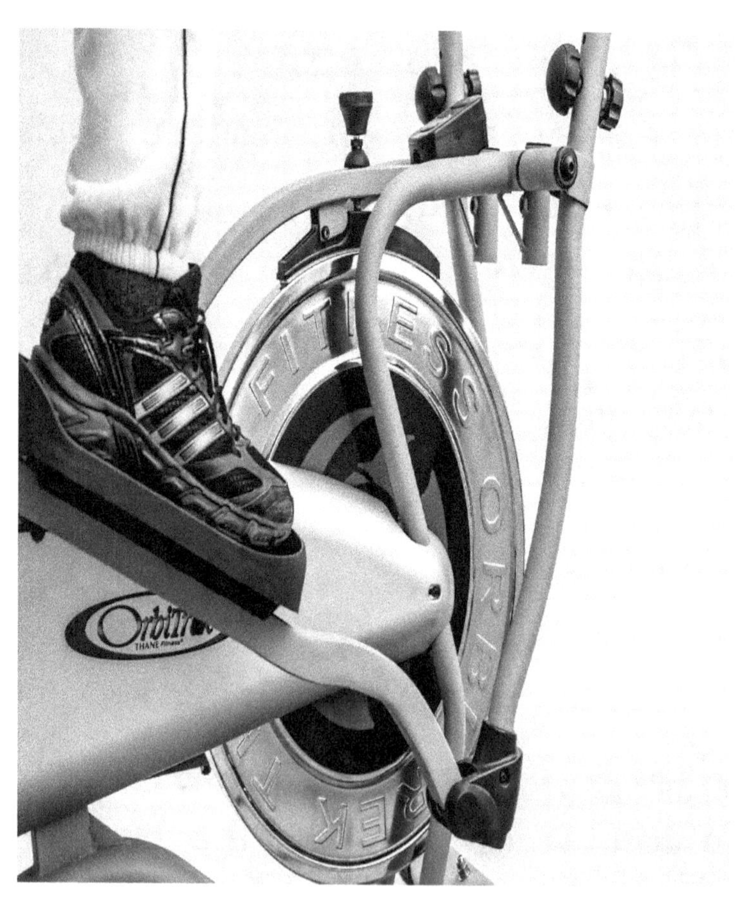

FITNESS ORBITREK

Sample Meal Plans & Grocery Lists

Consider an example shopping list and meal plan for a whole-body reset that focuses on managing weight loss. Please keep in mind that every person has different nutritional requirements, and it's wise to speak with a doctor or a nutritionist before making big dietary changes.

Meal Plan:

Day 1:

- **Breakfast:** Scrambled eggs with spinach and tomatoes
- **Mid-morning snack:** Greek yogurt with berries
- **Lunch:** Grilled chicken breast with quinoa and roasted vegetables
- **Afternoon snack:** Handful of almonds
- **Dinner:** Baked salmon with sweet potato and steamed broccoli.

Day 2:

- **Breakfast:** Oatmeal with sliced banana and a teaspoon of almond butter
- **Mid-morning snack:** Apple slices with a small portion of cheese
- **Lunch:** Turkey and avocado lettuce wraps with a side of cherry tomatoes
- **Afternoon snack:** Carrot sticks with hummus
- **Dinner:** Stir-fried tofu with mixed vegetables and brown rice.

Day 3:

- **Breakfast:** Smoothie with spinach, banana, almond milk, and protein powder
- **Mid-morning snack:** Cottage cheese with pineapple chunks
- **Lunch:** Quinoa salad with chickpeas, cucumber, and feta cheese
- **Afternoon snack:** Hard-boiled eggs with a sprinkle of black pepper
- **Dinner:** Grilled shrimp with asparagus and quinoa

Grocery List:

- **Proteins:**

Eggs

Chicken breast

Salmon

Tofu

Turkey

- **Grains:**

Quinoa

Brown rice

Oatmeal

- **Vegetables:**

Spinach

Tomatoes

Sweet potatoes

Broccoli

Lettuce

Avocado

Cherry tomatoes

Mixed vegetables (e.g., bell peppers, zucchini, carrots)

- **Fruits:**

Berries (blueberries, strawberries, raspberries)

Bananas

Apples

Pineapple

- **Dairy and Alternatives:**

Greek yogurt

Cheese

Almond milk

Cottage cheese

- **Nuts and Seeds:**

Almonds

Hummus

Chia seeds

- **Proteins (other):**

Shrimp

- **Pantry Staples:**

Olive oil (for cooking)

Almond butter

Whole-grain wraps

Always ensure to stay hydrated throughout the day and modify portion sizes according to your own energy requirements. This is only an example; you may adjust it to suit your nutritional needs and tastes.

Conclusion

The Whole Body Reset wasn't simply about dropping pounds (though we celebrated those successes!). It was about letting go of antiquated ideas, finding mobility again, and developing a strong connection between your body and mind. You conquered the beast of stress, discovered the power of real nourishment, and developed a growth-oriented, self-compassionate mentality.

You are now poised to live a life of true empowerment. What's next is as follows:

You've let go of self-doubt and accepted your health as a celebration rather than a burden. You now have a body you love and a mind you trust. Joyfully move your body, understanding that each stride is an investment in your future. Fill your cells with colorful, tasty food and enjoy the energy that propels your colorful existence.

A life without constraints and in rhythm: Give up dieting and adopt an intuitive eating style. Pay attention to your body's cues and act wisely—rather than deprived—in response. Allow movement to happen organically, driven by enthusiasm rather than guilt. Strive for balance in your life by giving sleep, self-care, and soul-nourishing activities first priority.

A rippling impact of transformation: Your path doesn't stop with you. Inspire everyone around you with your increased energy and confidence. Give your recipes, expertise, and passion for a well-balanced life a try. Be the catalyst for a whole-body wellness revolution in your neighborhood.

Reset was a catalyst, not a goal, so keep that in mind. You now possess the abilities and knowledge necessary to keep growing, overcome obstacles gracefully, and accept every turn, every victory, and every setback as a part of your unique and lovely journey.

Thus, reset warrior, advance with your head held high. The world is waiting for the happy ripple effect of your trip, your altered luminosity, and your irrepressible energy. Continue discovering, learning, and embracing your physical self. Move forth and lead your own reset.

This is your new beginning, your life, your metamorphosis. Take ownership of it, rejoice in it, and never stop telling your narrative with each attentive breath, wholesome decision, and mouthwatering mouthful. There are many options.

Beautiful person, shine on and go forward. The world is in need of your brightness.

www.ingramcontent.com/pod-product-compliance
Lightning Source LLC
Chambersburg PA
CBHW060945260726
48661CB00005B/1773